EAT CLEAN
and follow your
Dreams

D1508501

KELSEY BYERS

DEDICATION

This book is dedicated to my husband, Kent, who encouraged me to put my journey in writing. I love you. Thank you for being my best friend and number-one fan.

CONTENTS

ACKNOWLEDGMENTS

I am very thankful for the team of people that have stood by my side from the beginning of my journey. I am also thankful for those friends I have met along the way. I believe that God brings people together for a reason. I also believe that God never places a dream in your heart that He doesn't want you to pursue. He opens doors that no one else can and gives you the patience and discipline to see it through. God has guided and continues to guide my path every day. He has shown me how to use my abilities and knowledge to help others. He has shown me that my dreams are bigger than me, and I will be forever grateful for that.

Thank you to my husband, Kent, who encouraged me to "pick up" the weights and start lifting. He has supported my entire weight-loss journey and loves me for me. He is involved with every aspect of my career, and we are a team. I could not have made it this far without his love and support. We started this journey together, and I am thankful for his open mind and willingness to encourage my dreams. He is my best friend, chef, number-one fan, and the love of my life. I am so proud of how far we've come and can't wait to see what the future holds.

Thank you to my best friend, Diane, who has supported me on this journey of eating clean. She has never questioned my goals, even if she didn't always share or understand them. She has been such a loving and thoughtful friend, and I will never forget the friendship she has shown me. She is such a selfless person and shows kindness to everyone that comes in contact with her. She believed in my story enough to send my photos to *Oxygen Magazine,* which resulted in my first publication with *Oxygen* and hundreds of emails from others searching to find their way to a better body. Diane has transformed her own body and mind through adopting new healthy habits, and I've been blessed to be part of her journey.

Thank you to my nutritionist, Kim Porterfield, for showing me how to meet and exceed my goals. She must have thought I was crazy the day we met and I told her, "I want to be a fitness model." She just smiled and said, "This is what we need to do…" We put the plan into action, and I am so thankful for her knowledge and expertise in the field of nutrition. She is not only my nutritionist but a great friend and supporter.

I am thankful for Keith Klein, The Institute of Eating Management, and the blessings they bring to the lives of their clients. Their knowledge has shown my family how to eat clean and stay healthy for the rest of our lives.

Thank you to my family and friends who support my lifestyle. It is not always the easiest to understand, but I am thankful for their acceptance and love. My family knows I've always been a big dreamer, and I'm thankful for their understanding and support of my decision to do things my own way. I am very thankful to my parents for living by example and showing me how to work hard for what I want. I look forward to passing those lessons on to my own children one day.

Thank you to Team Labrada and Lee for supporting my journey and choosing me to be a sponsored athlete. I am very proud to be on such an inspirational team of people. We have a very special chemistry, and I am blessed to have such a strong support system through my Labrada family.

A special thank you to Jamie Eason. If it weren't for her willingness to respond to a fan's email a few years ago, I would not have found my nutritionist or be where I am today. It is because of her kindness that I will always set out to help at least one person every day. One response or one simple act of kindness can change someone's life.

INTRODUCTION

My journey is and always will be a work in progress. When I was beginning it, I searched everywhere for answers on how to lose weight. I never knew if what I was reading would actually work when I put it into practice, plus I was never really the "dieting" type. I could start a diet, but within a week I was bored and still had not seen results. Once I started getting results from clean eating, I vowed to myself that I would put my knowledge in one place in order to help others. I thought it would be a blog or website; I had no idea I would be inspired to write a book about it. By looking at my progress photos, there is no doubt that eating clean and lifting weights WORKS. I am even blown away by the photos. I look at my "before" photos and cannot believe that person is me. If I would not have lived the progress, I might be hesitant to believe just how SIMPLE it is to lose weight the healthy way and *keep* it off.

The words you are about to read explain the process and lifestyle change that I went through in order to achieve the physique of my dreams. I not only lost the weight, but I work hard each day to maintain a healthy and fit body. I want to share the knowledge that I have learned that got me to this point of loving my body and improving my self-confidence. I owe much of my success to my nutritionist, Kim Porterfield, who not only taught me how to meet and exceed my goals but how to maintain a healthy body for the rest of my life. Her knowledge and encouragement changed my way of viewing food as fuel, not entertainment. She changed my life, and I will be forever grateful.

If you want to change your lifestyle, YOU have to be ready. There is no magic pill. My transformation was due to continuously motivating myself, even when results were not coming as quickly as I'd hoped. I will tell you this: the way to transform your body in the healthiest and quickest way possible is to eat clean. Plain and simple. No diet will help you lose weight and keep it off. If I had known about the value of a clean meal plan sooner, I could have lost my weight years earlier. However, I believe that there is a reason for everything, and God has a plan for my story.

Once you hit rock bottom and get fed up with the person you see in the mirror, you start searching for a way to change. You can become desperate. This is often the point people are at when I receive emails from them. Just know that clean eating is the answer, and if you practice smart habits consistently, the weight will fall off faster—I promise. The good news is time flies by. Before you know it, you will feel like a new person inside and out. Within three to four months of clean eating, my body completely reshaped itself. How long do you have to eat clean? Well, that all depends on how long you want to look and feel great. Let's get started.

Kelsey Byers
Houston, Texas, 2012

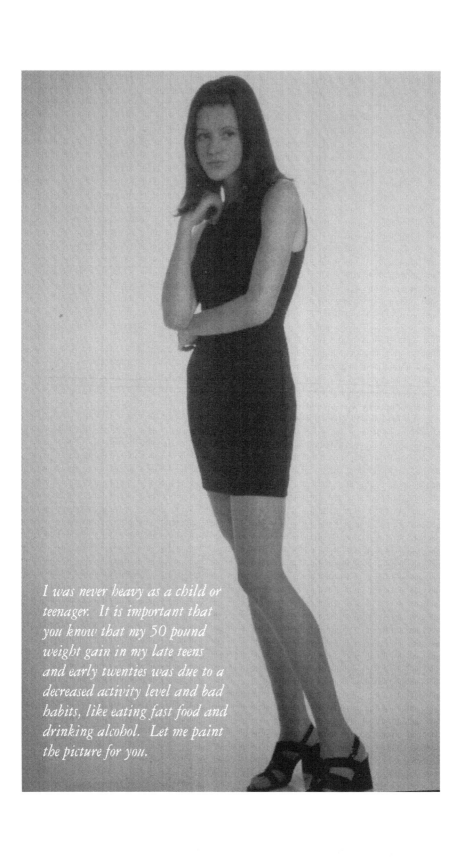

I was never heavy as a child or teenager. It is important that you know that my 50 pound weight gain in my late teens and early twenties was due to a decreased activity level and bad habits, like eating fast food and drinking alcohol. Let me paint the picture for you.

Chapter 1

STRING BEAN

I want to give you a brief insight on what it was like growing up a string bean. It is interesting what you can get away with eating when you are thirteen to seventeen years old, before your body really understands what you are putting in it. My body decided to give me a few years of "fun food" before it decided to grab on to fifty pounds and hold on for dear life. Here we go.

I grew up in the small town of Normangee, Texas. There was one flashing stop light, one small grocery store, a bank, a café, and a few gas stations. I believe the population sign read "seven hundred." My mom grew up there, too. Her dad was the town mayor for over twenty years, and everyone in town knew our family. My mom met my dad in Houston after college, then they moved back to Normangee once my sister and I were born. My dad started a successful air-conditioning business and my mom was a school teacher. She was even my teacher for a few classes once I got into junior high and high school. If I misbehaved in school, my mom knew about it by the next class period. I didn't get away with much in school.

I went from kindergarten through high school with most of the same kids. There were ups and downs to growing up in a small town. Everyone knew your business and what you did last weekend. The classes were smaller than those in a larger school, so students got more attention. There wasn't much to do entertainment-wise.

The nearest mall or movie theater was about thirty miles away, so my sister and I spent a lot of time outdoors. The Internet was not used much in our high school except for school projects, and there was no social networking. At age sixteen, my first vehicle was a dark-blue, single-cab GMC pickup truck. I loaded up as many friends as I could inside and we would make the "block" in town after school. This means we would crank up the radio and drive on one road that surrounds the town. We thought it was fun, and all the high school kids did it. We thought we were so cool!

I played as many sports as I could in junior high and high school. Since my mom was a teacher and loved sports, I had little choice but to be involved. Plus, I liked being active. At five-ten and 134 pounds, I played basketball, volleyball, track, cross country, golf, and was a dance team officer. I ate exactly what I wanted but didn't slow down long enough to gain weight. If I wasn't at dance team practice, I was practicing some other sport.

Even after basketball practice, most days I would go home and work out again. I would go running, shoot hoops in our driveway, or do crunches. It's not that I was obsessed, but these were before the days of social networking, so I had to keep myself from getting bored. Growing up in the country on sixteen acres, my sister and I weren't too into watching TV, so we kept ourselves entertained outdoors.

We fished, rode four-wheelers, and raised chickens in 4-H, an agricultural club at school. I believe that growing up in a small town and juggling many activities at once is what led me to be the multi-tasker I am today. Our upbringing wasn't any different than my classmates' so I looked at it as normal. Once I got to college and told new friends about my childhood, I realized just how special and unique growing up in a small town was. That is something I would never want to change.

We were one busy family. My dad worked really hard to support us and our many activities. With his air-conditioning business, he was always working in the heat, so I'm sure he burned plenty of calories at work. My mom stayed active, too. She worked full time, as well as running my sister and me all over town to our extracurricular activities. Once I could drive, I'm sure my mom was on the go less but probably worried a little more.

I always remember her eating fairly healthy and walking our fence line on our property for exercise. My family was never heavy, so we didn't think we needed to change our eating habits. My mom prepared balanced meals at night for dinner. When I tell you I could eat anything and get away with it, I do mean anything. My sister and I ate Eggo waffles or Pop Tarts every morning for breakfast for years. I would drink about three glasses of whole milk a day.

I could eat fried chicken fingers and a baked potato loaded in ranch dressing for lunch at school then go home and eat Velveeta shells and cheese at dinner. I didn't think I was eating unhealthily—I didn't think about it at all. It was normal.

I would eat my vegetables every night with dinner, so I thought that was healthy enough. My favorite fast food was a cheeseburger from Sonic with extra mayonnaise, along with tater tots covered in melted cheese. Since we didn't have a Sonic in Normangee, fast food was a special occasion when we were out of town. At sixteen years old, I started working for a local country club as a waitress in the restaurant. I would order food off of the menu and chow down, guilt-free. By now you get the point that my weight was not a problem for me in high school.

I tell you this little bit of history so you will understand what a shock I was in for just a few short years later. I vowed to myself that when I graduated high school, I would join a gym, promising myself that I would never get fat. Upon graduation from high school, I weighed about 134 pounds and wore a size four in pants and dresses. I could not wait to move out and go to college. The world was mine for the taking! I felt like I knew it all. I wanted to start fresh where no one knew me or my family. I just wanted to create myself.

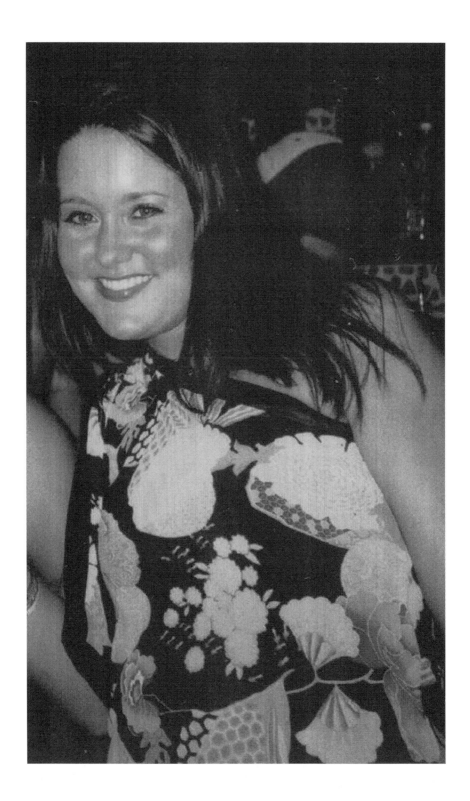

Chapter 2

CHUNKY COLLEGE CHICK

Upon graduating, I moved out as soon as I could. I had the entire summer to get settled and find a job. I was so excited to have responsibility and my own freedom. I moved thirty miles away to the nearest college town and enrolled in my basic college classes. I moved into a one-bedroom condo by myself. This was my first time living alone. I got a job at a grocery store deli, slicing lunch meat and making sandwiches and fruit trays. If I wasn't eating sandwiches and snacks from the store deli and bakery, I was eating ramen noodles. They were simple and cheap.

It wasn't that I couldn't afford anything else; I just wasn't sure what to cook. I had never been on my own and usually didn't stay at my condo long enough to plan a good meal, so I would eat quick, easy meals or drive in for fast food. My pants started getting tight. I was living life and enjoying every aspect of being social and hanging out with friends.

After a few months went by, I found a new job as a medical receptionist. The pay was better, and I wasn't constantly surrounded by food anymore. Most of my new coworkers were college kids my age. We would order fast food for delivery at lunch and all meet up after work for happy hour.

I slowly started "filling out" and had to buy new clothes. I applied for my first credit card so I could go shopping for new clothes. I'm sure I told myself I needed new, more stylish clothes, but, truth be told, I couldn't fit into my old ones. I also wore scrubs at my new job, so it wasn't as noticeable that I was gaining weight. Slowly but surely, my clothes sizes started increasing. I started college in a size four and, within a year, I was in a size eight. Size eight would have been a healthy size to stay in, but that apparently wasn't a wake-up call for me.

Another year went by and I was wearing sizes ten to twelve. I suppose I was waiting for someone to stop me and tell me I was fat. To stop my new found bad habits. To make some changes and get my body healthy. No one ever did. Gaining weight and living an on-the-go lifestyle was actually the norm for the college students I surrounded myself with. I was a social butterfly who loved going dancing, drinking, and eating. I loved every minute of it. I just didn't love who I saw in the mirror anymore.

A bigger milestone soon came about: I turned twenty-one. Being from a small town and not having much to do, I had already experienced my share of alcoholic beverages. However, the age of twenty-one brought new freedom and social excitement I had never felt before. I could go to restaurants and order delicious drinks at dinner. Even if I wanted to eat something slightly healthy, as soon as I started drinking, it would cause me to reach for anything to snack on. I was going out two or three nights a week with my friends, eating junk food late at night, getting little sleep, going to work, then repeating.

I developed a really low self-esteem and bad body image. I dreaded the thought of trying on swimsuits and conveniently found other things to do when a pool party was going on. As much as I liked to party and be social, I did not want anyone seeing me in a swimsuit. By this point, I had gained about thirty-five to forty pounds. I was dating, but the relationships were dramatic, centered around the partying lifestyle, and my low self-esteem left me little room for confidence. To say I was unhappy was an understatement.

My grades in college were "okay" considering I wasn't giving my school work much priority. I had no idea what I wanted to do in life, so it was tough trying to figure that out and focus on college while maintaining an active social life and working part time. By this point, my younger female cousin had graduated from Normangee high school and moved to the same college town. We were very close throughout high school, and I was overjoyed to have her living close by. I imagine I was a bad influence on her at some point. I was the oldest and had been in college a year before her.

I remember her making the comment one day that she did not want to drink during the week because that was "way too many calories." I remember thinking that was the silliest thing I had ever heard. Why would you risk not having "fun" so you wouldn't consume the calories? I didn't get it. My cousin is tall and beautiful, hitting the six-foot mark. She maintained a lean physique in college and the "freshman fifteen" stayed away from her.

I remember going out dancing with her, and all of the guys flocked to her. She was never hurting for attention. We loved getting dressed up and going out together. Over time, the guys quit noticing me. At first I thought it was because they were intimidated. I laugh now thinking about it. As time went by, I realized they just were not interested. For some reason, they just weren't even attracted. My beloved cousin did not experience this same problem.

Her body was still lean, just as it was in high school. We were both eating the same things when we were together, so I did not understand why I continued to gain weight but she didn't. It wasn't that I felt jealous; she was my best friend. However, I did wonder what I was missing. Until this point, I had never craved attention or felt the need to be complimented. I was always confident and carefree. But at this point in my life, I was craving compliments, attention, and a thinner body.

I had a gym membership, so I would go and complete forty-five-minute cardio sessions on the elliptical a few days a week. I would feel so proud of myself when I was done. I would finish that job well done with a night drinking and eating pizza with friends. I was right in the middle of a vicious cycle. Looking back, I had no idea that nutrition played such a big part in the way I looked.

I now believe that nutrition makes up 80 percent of the way you look, the other 20 percent being exercise. In my workouts, I was sticking to cardio only and was not confident when it came to lifting weights with proper form. I had no idea which exercise worked which muscle group.

I had developed an addiction to shopping. If I saw women out and about who looked really cute, I would search for those same outfits, hoping I would look the same way. I was miserable. No outfit gave me the feeling of confidence that I was after. I would watch my cousin when we went out together. She seemed confident, free-spirited, and definitely not worrying about her outfit.

I, on the other hand, was always tugging and pulling at whatever I had on. Nothing fit right, nor was it comfortable. The more depressed I got about it, the more alcohol I wanted to drink when we would go out.

Alcohol made me temporarily confident. It made me feel like I didn't care, and being out drinking was the only time I could "escape from myself." What I didn't realize at the time is that alcohol is a depressant. Not only was it making me fatter, it was making me even more depressed about it. I was drinking, getting hungry, and snacking on fast food.

Out of all my friends, I was the one who carried a camera around. I was constantly snapping photos. I loved to scrapbook and made a book for each year of college. When I was at my heaviest, I started just snapping pictures of others and realized that I did not want to be photographed with them. I am so glad some of my friends insisted on my being in the pictures. Little did I know we were capturing my "before" photos that have motivated so many people to lose weight having seen my transformation!

One morning after waking up with a headache from drinking all night, I started going through clothes in my closet. I'm sure I was wondering what I would wear out that night. I noticed that the sizes in my closet ranged from a size four to a size twelve-fourteen. I could not believe I let myself get to that point. The weight came on so fast that I had not even taken the time to clean out my closet. I'm thankful for that now.

I had never been one to weigh myself, but I walked across the street to the gym near my condo. I stepped on the scale and was completely shocked that I weighed 176 pounds. Somewhere in that two-year time frame, I gained a total of about forty-five pounds. You see, no one stopped me and had an intervention. No one told me I was living unhealthily. No one told me I was heading down the road to obesity.

I was starting to get winded when climbing stairs at school. I would get tired really quickly when I went out dancing with friends. We would always joke that going dancing was our cardio. What I was actually doing was cardio, but I was dehydrating myself with one alcoholic drink after another. The combination of the new weight I was carrying with little sleep, bad nutrition, and alcohol was taking its toll on me.

One night, the switch of motivation in my head flipped on. I was hanging out with a guy friend at my condo. I was watching TV, and he was going through voicemails on his cell phone. He had the speaker volume up, so I could faintly hear the messages. I heard another male friend's familiar voice on a message. He said, "Hey, man! Where have you been? You must be hanging out with that WHALE again." The message stopped me dead in my tracks. A sick feeling started to form in my stomach.

I asked my friend, "Who have you been hanging out with? That was so rude of him to say about someone." My friend laughed and tried to change the subject, but I was not budging. After several more minutes of questioning, he finally admitted, "He was talking about YOU." I was stunned.

I'm sure I was not great company the rest of that evening because all I could do was replay the words in my head: "that WHALE." All through high school, I was a thin and athletic size four. Clothes always looked good and felt good on me. I had never hurt in the attention department from guys. Now, here was this guy I had considered a friend calling me names and referring to me as fat. Talk about a huge reality check.

I looked in the mirror and knew I needed a change. I needed to change for me, not anyone else. Not for attention, not to wear smaller clothes or look good in photos. For me. I needed to get healthy. Enough was enough. Not only was I sick of looking at myself in the mirror; I was tired of some of the company I was keeping. Who wants to be around "friends" who make you feel negative inside? I knew the change needed to start within me first.

I knew I had to be happy with myself before I could expect to have a fulfilling relationship. I decided to transfer colleges and start over fresh. I also decided I wanted to change my major from biology to business. I was starting to think about my future and wanted a degree in the business field. I moved to a new town and separated myself from most of the crowd I partied with. I assumed we would all stay friends and would still make an effort to hang out. I only moved fifty miles away. The truth is we rarely saw each other after that, signaling to me that our "friendships" were built around a lifestyle instead of an actual relationship. I would call and leave messages scheduling to get together, but slowly the relationships faded.

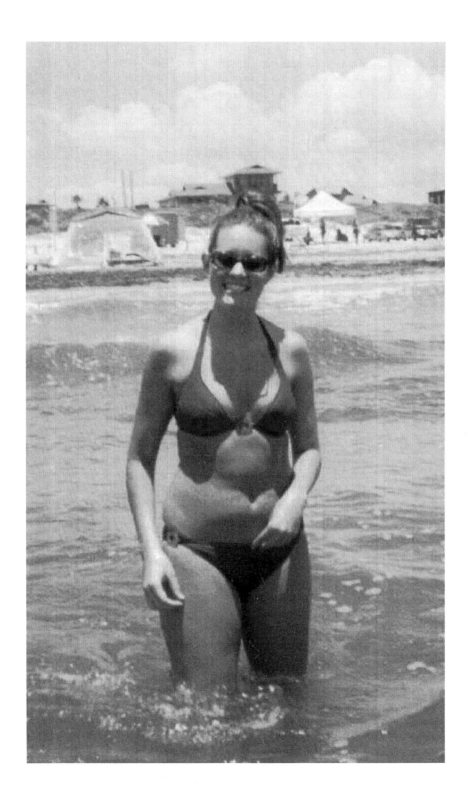

Chapter 3

MOTIVATION: COURAGE TO CHANGE

Once I started back to school the following semester, I hired a female trainer at our college recreation center. She taught me proper form with lifting and suggested I start writing down what I ate throughout the day in order to track my progress. A few months later, I met my future husband, Kent. I can't tell you it was love at first sight.

We met while we were out one night with some mutual friends. Before we met, my friend told me, "You will love Kent. He's perfect. He doesn't drink or smoke and works out all the time. He even goes to church." It was all true and, it turns out, he was perfect for me. However, we did not officially start dating until nine months later when we saw each other again at a graduation party. I was still trying to find that balance of socializing on a smaller scale and giving school more focus. Kent was very built and muscular. On our second date, a waiter asked him how big his biceps were. After spending more time with him, I realized he was the most disciplined person I had ever met. He simply liked to work out to feel good.

I was immediately impressed with Kent's discipline for saying no to sweets and processed foods. The first time he met my mom, she offered him one of her homemade chocolate chip cookies. He politely declined and said, "No, thank you, I don't eat refined sugar." You can imagine the look on my mom's face. She must have looked at me like, "WHO have you brought home?" She was impressed with anyone's ability to turn down her homemade cookies.

Kent's outlook on food was something I had never encountered before. At that point, I had not even brushed the surface of what real self-discipline was. For so long, I had grown accustomed to the idea of instant gratification. If I craved something, I thought I needed it right then and there, whether it was food, alcohol, shopping, you name it.

I had no real concept of the benefits of delayed gratification—for example, eating healthy now to create a healthy body, saving money for my future, and so on. I had to learn a very tough lesson on what delayed gratification meant. I slowly started changing my habits. I began working out with Kent, and he strongly encouraged me to start lifting weights. Up until that point, my workouts consisted mainly of cardio. I had little knowledge on what to do in the weight room, other than bench presses and what my trainer had demonstrated.

Kent started teaching me proper form with lifting and showed me which exercises targeted different muscle groups. Within just a few short months of lifting, I could see more definition in my arms and legs. He encouraged me to start lifting heavy. Kent explained to me that women are not made up the way men are and would need more testosterone to get bulky. I think most women are afraid they will bulk up. Kent's point was that weights would tone me and give my body a new shape. At this point, I was fluctuating between sizes ten and twelve, down from a size fourteen. I was making progress.

I made my weight-loss goals clear to Kent, and he was very supportive. I didn't necessarily want to be the same size I was in high school, but I wanted to feel good in my clothes. We started cooking at my apartment more and going out to eat less. I avoided alcohol and was surprisingly able to cut it out of my diet for a month straight during one semester.

I was shocked at how easy it was to avoid alcohol when my lifestyle didn't center around going out to parties or clubs and staying out late. I discovered I had just as much fun sober, hanging out with friends, going bowling, taking trips, and going to the gym. Within the next year, I graduated college, and Kent and I got engaged. We had a year-long engagement and, by the day of our wedding, I was in a size eight wedding dress. That weight loss was due to trial and error, avoiding alcohol, and going out to eat less. I felt confident and beautiful on the day of our wedding. My dress was beautiful and fit perfectly. Kent and I bought a house and moved to the Houston area. It was then that I started a new job behind a desk and joined a new gym.

One day on my lunch break, my best friend, Diane, and I noticed a fitness model's photo on MySpace. She was this fit, muscular, beautiful blonde with an amazing physique. THAT was my turning point. The model's name is Jamie Eason. She was the first person who made muscle look beautiful to me. I suddenly desired to have the fit physique of an athlete. I got the nerve to email her the next day through MySpace. She surprisingly responded with plenty of encouragement and tips on how to get fit. Her number-one piece of advice was: hire a nutritionist.

At the time, Jamie lived in Houston, too, so she referred me to the nutritionist's office where she first learned about CLEAN

EATING. That was my introduction. My body was definitely achieving results from lifting weights, but I wanted to take it to the next level. Kent wasn't too thrilled about the idea of paying someone to tell him how to eat. After all, we ate "healthy" anyway. At least we thought we did. I took a running total of how much money we spent going out to eat each month and finally convinced him to use that money to visit a nutritionist. What we did not realize at the time is that our lives would soon change.

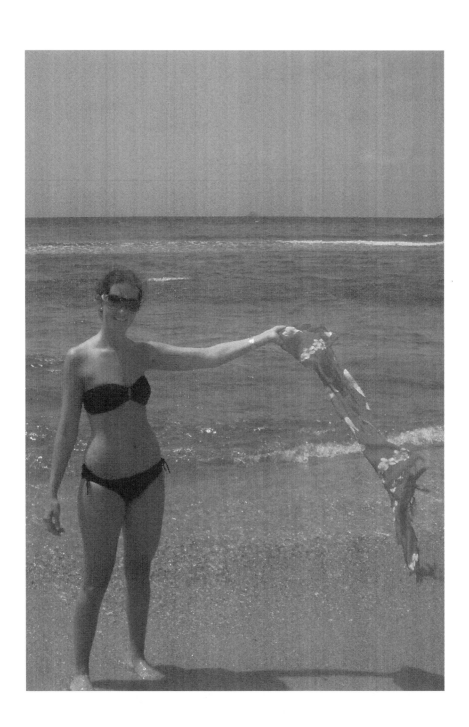

Chapter 4

NUTRITIONIST

When I called the Institute of Eating Management, I decided I would like to visit the female nutritionist on staff. I remember telling her that I wanted to hire someone who "practices what they preach." She told me that I had come to the right place. She was a former figure competitor and personal trainer. I had this feeling that she was the perfect person to help me achieve my goals.

At our first office visit with our nutritionist, she took our body weight, body fat, and noted our eating habits. The good news is that Kent and I were not too far off with our eating habits; we simply needed customized measured portions. Our nutritionist asked us our goals. We both explained that we wanted more energy to fuel our workouts in the gym. Kent's goal was to lean out in his mid-section.

When it came my turn to announce my goal, I spoke from my heart and told the truth, no matter how ridiculous I thought it would sound: "I want to be a fitness model." I still remember my nutritionist's facial expression to this day. She was probably expecting me to say that I wanted to lose ten pounds, have fit abs, look good in a swimsuit, something "normal." The truth is I have wanted to model since the age of twelve. My mom sent my sister and me to modeling school but, living far from the city, it was tough to get to jobs.

My mom always told me to finish high school and college then encouraged me to do whatever I wanted. My dad always told me, "You can be anything you want; just apply yourself." This was me ready to apply myself. In my mind, this was my chance. At twenty-eight years old, I knew that most fitness models were in their thirties, so I believed it was perfect timing.

My nutritionist customized meal plans for Kent and me, and we immediately got started. We started eating every three hours, five to seven meals a day. I had read in different magazines that this was the key to earning a lean body, and the visit to our nutritionist confirmed that it was true. We were ready to put our plan into action.

It was tough preparing all of the food at first, but once we created the habit, it was second nature. Starting out, we would indulge in cheat meals occasionally, once every two weeks. This was a step up from our previous once-a-week cheat meals. We went to our nutrition visit follow-ups every two weeks, so she could tell if we had been following her plan or cheating. That provided a new level of accountability. Here we were, paying a professional to teach us how to eat, so we decided to buckle down and really stick with it.

When we hired our nutritionist, Kent and I both had body fat percentages at 24 percent. I've read that women are considered healthy in the 20 to 25 percent range and men in the 10 to 15 percent range. While my body fat was finally healthy again since college, I still had this strong motivation to take my body to the next level. Kent felt the same way. We were both experiencing low energy levels in the gym and were certain that our portion sizes had something to do with it. It turns out we were under-eating prior to our nutritionist visit. Both under-eating and over-eating can cause your body to hold on to unwanted fat.

I would like to point out that the beginning of my weight-loss journey was the hardest. It is natural to want results right now and get discouraged after not seeing any after one week of clean eating and lifting weights. Remember that everyone's body is unique and responds differently to food. It took about two months of clean eating before my body's metabolism kicked into high gear.

I had never eaten that much in my life, much less measure my portions. I thought it seemed a little extreme, but if Jamie Eason said it worked, there had to be something to it. It didn't take long before my body was telling me when it was time to eat. Around the two-and-a-half-hour mark, my stomach would start growling. My body loved the clean meals and used the food as fuel for my workouts in the gym. Not only did I have more energy, my body's shape started changing.

My arms became more defined and the weight I held around my waist and hips slowly started disappearing. When I hired my nutritionist, I weighed 140 pounds and had 24 percent body fat. After just four months of clean eating, I had gotten down to 15 percent body fat, still weighing 140 pounds. I'm glad I wasn't fixed on the scale because my weight never changed. I had simply replaced fat with muscle.

Muscle weighs the same as fat; it just takes up less room. Muscle transforms your body into a tight little package that looks great in anything: clothing, swimsuits, anything. Kent was down to 8 percent body fat, which was a huge difference from 24 percent just months earlier. For me, the best part of all was when I got down to 15 percent body fat—the cellulite that was once on the back of my legs almost disappeared completely.

Before I started eating clean, I had already accepted the fact that my cellulite would never go away. I just thought it was genetics or maybe my body just held fat there. However, by eliminating processed foods and extra sugar from my diet, the fat slowly disappeared and the cellulite followed! I was thrilled with my results.

We went from being a normal-looking couple on the beach to a fit and firm dynamic duo. Perfect strangers started approaching us in the gym and grocery store, asking what we did. The biggest misconception of all is that people assumed we spent hours in the gym every day. When we told them it was mostly food, they looked relieved but doubtful. We were consistently working out in the gym for one hour, five days a week, getting lean and replacing fat with muscle.

Kent and I decided to attend a fitness competition one weekend just to see what it was about. As I watched the fit ladies in the bikini division take the stage, a new motivation transpired. My wheels were turning. During our next nutrition follow-up visit, my body was still 15 percent body fat.

My nutritionist explained to me that I was considered in the athletic body fat percentage range and that I could easily start training for a competition. I think all I needed was that encouragement. Shortly after our visit, I chose a show and committed to a twelve-week training program. We talked about my plan and what it would require me to add to my routine. There were also things I would need to avoid, like alcohol and cheat meals. I thought to myself, *I can do anything for twelve weeks. That's only three months.* A week later, training began.

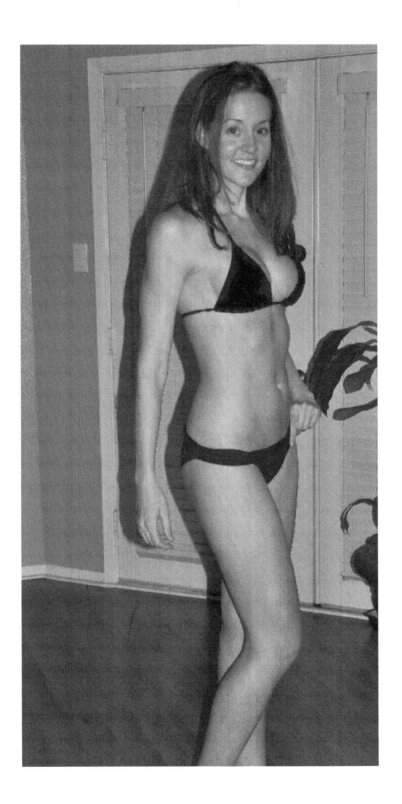

Chapter 5

BIKINI COMPETITOR

As you can see from my journey so far, my transformation wasn't overnight. I slowly morphed into this disciplined, motivated, positive person. I knew and accepted the fact that big changes would not occur overnight, so I found small things to keep me motivated along the way. At one point, I started a photo album on my home computer filled with photos of my favorite fitness models, athletes, and motivational quotes.

When I started training for my first NPC (National Physique Committee) bikini competition, I cut out alcohol completely. I avoided going out to eat because I did not know how the food would be cooked or what butter and oils they would use. The twelve weeks tested and tempted me more than I could ever imagine. There is something about telling yourself, "Don't do this," that makes you want it more.

I won't pretend I didn't have a single cheat meal or drink of alcohol in those whole twelve weeks. I probably had five slip-ups total. I had a couple glasses of wine and gave in to peanut butter and chocolate at some point. On a trip with my family, I successfully avoided my mom's homemade chocolate chip cookies for three days.

On the fourth day, a hungry monster in my head told me to eat one. I ate one, and one turned to five. I felt miserable for caving in, but I only had myself to answer to. I decided then and there that this was MY goal and I needed to stay on track. I will also say that I worked harder on my training in the gym during those twelve weeks than ever before in my life.

Actually placing and winning a trophy did not cross my mind. I was simply going to prove to myself that I had the nerve and the body to get on stage in front of hundreds of people. To be honest, the thought of being compared to beautiful women based entirely on my physique terrified me. I just knew that people would be able to see every little dimple and flaw under those bright lights. Still, I knew I had come this far and had a small support group that encouraged me on a daily basis. I kept pushing forward.

I followed up with visits to my nutritionist every two weeks to track my weight and body fat percentage. About a month before the show, I almost chickened out. There was still a spot of cellulite on my left leg that would not budge. I broke down and cried to my husband in the kitchen one night and told him I did not feel like my results were "enough" to get on stage.

Kent reassured me that I looked great, but even he had no idea what a competitor should look like at this point in training. At our next appointment, my nutritionist explained to me that four weeks for a competitor was plenty of time to meet my goals. My husband still encouraged me, making the point that I had worked so hard to get to this level. They were right. I decided to continue with my training. I had to do this for ME. I think it's normal to doubt yourself. There were moments that "Chunky Kelsey" still took over my brain and I could not believe it was actually my body I saw in the mirror.

My body was transforming so fast before my eyes that my mind could not keep up. I saw new, small changes every day, so this kept me pushing forward. I was waking up five to six days a week for morning cardio and lifting weights at night. I was eating every three hours like clockwork. I felt like a fat-burning machine.

I had never been that lean and muscular in my life. I felt really strong, too. I ate a lean protein and complex carbohydrate at each meal. The beauty of training is that I didn't feel like I was dieting, just avoiding junk food and alcohol. For the first time in my life, I was eating only what my body needed.

One of the fun parts of competing is choosing your suit. It's important to choose one that complements you. I decided to buy two bikinis, just to have a backup. I bought my required clear high heels and practiced posing. I even hired someone to teach me in a posing class to get pointers on stage presence.

I walked around in those heels for weeks preparing for my show. I arranged to have my spray tan done the night before the competition. Your tan should be dark enough to bring out your definition on stage. Under the bright lights, it looks normal next to the other competitors. However, in person, you look orange.

At my final appointment the week of my show, my nutritionist informed me that I had met my goal of 10 percent body fat. That meant I had achieved 50 percent of my goal! Now I just had to take the stage. It was such an incredible feeling of empowerment. My nutritionist gave me the last instructions before the show and off I went.

The rest of the week was a blur. I've heard some competitors call it "diet head" when you feel like you are in a "dream land" state. Your body is stripped down and lean. You can usually only maintain the lean body fat percentage for a few weeks. After that, it's healthy and wise to get back to your normal routine and introduce healthy fats and more carbohydrates back into your system. This prevents your hormones from being imbalanced.

My competition day arrived and I checked in at the front of the venue with all of my food for the day. I arrived in my bikini wearing a jumpsuit over it. The day was quite long and the bikini division was the last to compete. The athletes were required to check in early—hurry up and wait. Trust me, that gives you plenty of time to doubt yourself.

Luckily, I had met my goals so far, so I felt pretty confident. I remember being backstage with the other competitors before prejudging. This was the first time I was side by side with other women training for the same goal as myself. I remember thinking, *I kind of look like these ladies.* I was perfectly happy with my results and already felt like a winner. I had achieved something even when my mind told me, *You could never do that.* I had succeeded.

I met many nice people at the show; we even shared craving and clean eating tips backstage. I was in the tallest height class because I am five-ten. While waiting to line up, I took my jumpsuit off and put my high heels on. I quickly noticed that my spray tan had stained the bottoms of my white suit. It was ruined and the stain would be obvious on stage. I quickly changed into my backup suit. Good thing I went prepared!

I was surprisingly even more confident in my backup suit than in my original choice. The backup was white with black zebra stripes and was lined in red lace. Very sassy. I got so many compliments on that suit. The moment arrived for me to take the stage. I had about fifteen seconds to impress the judges.

Each competitor wore a number pinned to her suit, which helped the judges identify us. I walked out on stage with a big smile on my face. I went through the motions of the posing I had practiced time and time again. I was just praying that I did not fall and make a fool of myself. My heart was racing, and I hoped the judges and the crowd could not tell I was shaking from the adrenaline. The energy of being on stage was captivating, and I felt strong and confident.

I had achieved 100 percent of my goal. I walked on that stage at 10 percent body fat, which was the perfect look for my body type. I even made it across the stage in my high heels without falling. What more could I ask for? Once I walked off stage, I remember the announcer calling the top five numbers for first callout.

That usually means you placed in the top five, but you don't actually find out until the evening show. The announcer called my number! I remember checking and rechecking the number pinned on my suit to make sure they were calling me. I walked back onstage with four other women for a comparison lineup. I could not believe it.

Once it was time for the finals that night, there was a surprise in store for me. I not only walked on stage for the evening show— I placed third in my bikini height class, qualified for nationals, and went home with a trophy! I was amazed that I was able to train myself in the gym and meet my goals with the help of my nutritionist in just a few short months. It just goes to show that nutrition makes up so much of the way you look.

It wasn't actually until I looked at my photos a month after the show that I realized how lean I had gotten. My journey to the stage was the hardest I have ever worked at anything in my life. This time in my life strengthened my relationship with God. I found myself praying about everything: praying for discipline, for motivation, for patience, for strength, you name it.

Any time I had self-doubt based on someone else's comments and opinions, I prayed. It was during that time that God gave me the strength to keep going. Any time I doubted my actions and my purpose for competing, something positive would happen that would strongly support my decision to continue. I didn't know any other competitors, so I really had no one to compare myself to other than the athletes I researched on the Internet. It really was quite remarkable what a clean meal plan and consistent training did for my body.

The hardest part during that journey was saying no to the temptations I was accustomed to saying yes to—for example, wine, sushi, peanut butter, and going out to eat. Another obstacle I experienced was that not everyone around me really understood my goal. Not everyone realized how much weight I had actually lost at this point, so they made comments about my goal being about vanity. My weight loss was gradual and took place over about a five-year period.

What the naysayers did not realize is that the very goal of competing was my proof to myself that I could overcome any obstacle, particularly the bad habits with food and alcohol that had built up over the course of a few years. I was fighting every day to create new habits. I was teaching myself a new lifestyle, and my "graduation" was the day I walked on that stage.

Your body is like a science experiment in a way. When you fuel it with the right foods, the right training, and rest, you can achieve any goal you set. Once you get past the idea of looking at food as entertainment, you can do wonders for your body and your mind. You finally feel in control. After my competition, I felt empowered that I could go after any goal.

It was then that I decided to enroll in graduate school to earn my master's degree in business administration, something I had wanted to do for six years. Achieving my personal fitness goals flipped a switch in my head. I was no longer the same woman who gave up on goals. I knew if I made up my mind, I could achieve anything. I was learning how to let my discipline in one area of life spill into the other areas. I felt renewed.

As far as competing goes, I didn't go to nationals in 2010 because my husband and I were not prepared for the expense of it. Again, that tells you I never planned to place—I simply wanted to walk the stage. I had not given any thought to the question, "What's next?" I didn't even know I qualified for nationals until I walked off stage with my trophy and another competitor said, "Congratulations on qualifying for nationals." Competing is an expensive sport once you factor in hotel costs, spray tan, bathing suit, food, nutrition, training, and more. It was time to figure out my path in fitness, and I needed some time to figure that out.

Not long after my competition, I was contacted by Labrada Nutrition in Houston. They invited me to represent their brand as an athlete and shoot for their summer catalogue. My husband and I were already using Labrada's Lean Body Meal Replacement shakes, so I quickly accepted their invitation to represent their brand and to become a sponsored athlete. I have learned since that it is most competitors' goal to be sponsored to compete. I am extremely grateful for the opportunity that was presented to me by Labrada Nutrition so early on in my fitness career.

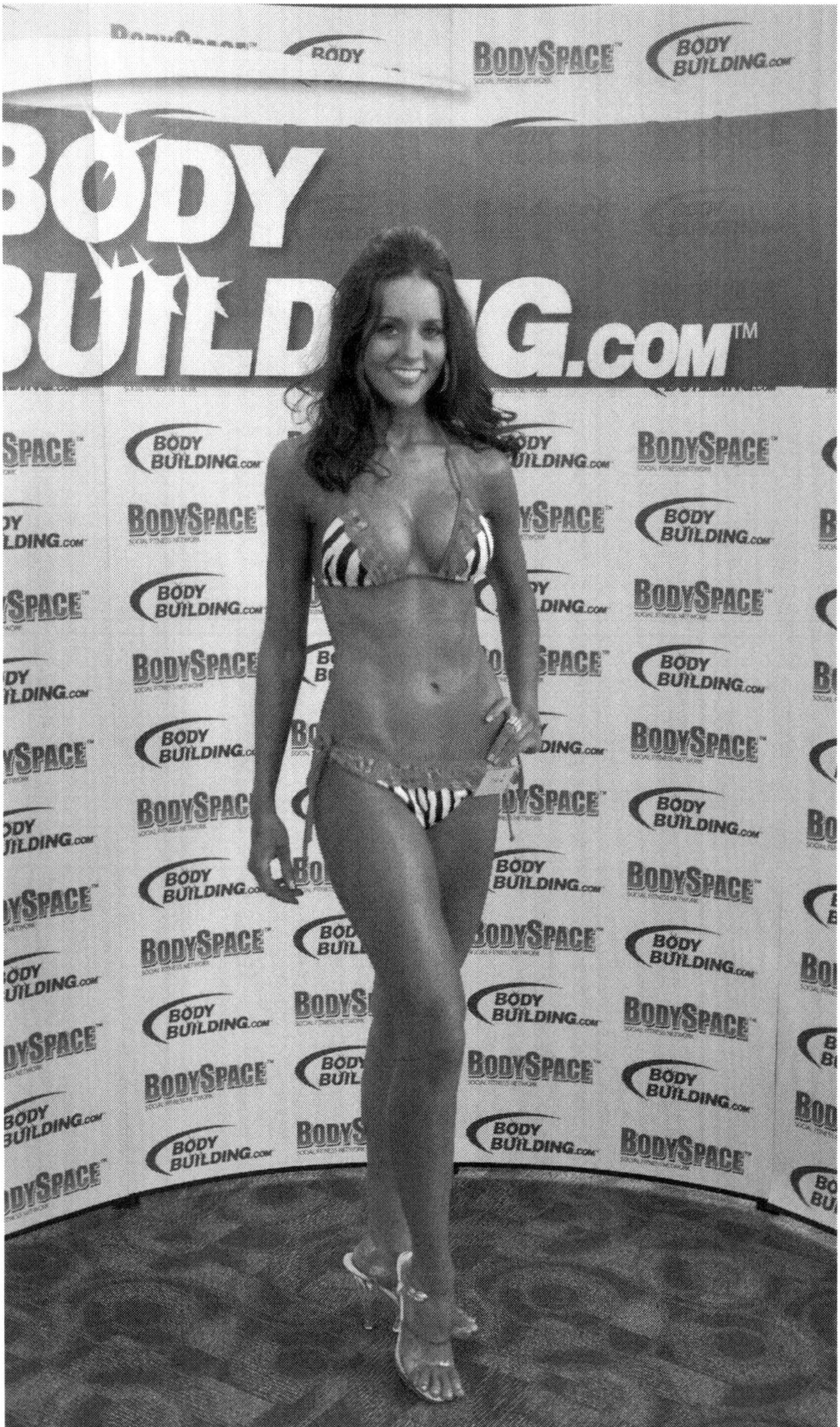

Chapter 6

POST-COMPETITION

It is important that I include this chapter to follow competing. I don't want you to think that I competed and stayed in tip-top shape from that point on. That would be misleading. Like I mentioned before, there is something about telling yourself NO for twelve weeks then, all of a sudden, you can tell yourself YES. That hungry monster in my head was set free!

I actually had a running list of the foods I wanted to eat post-competition. This list included various sweets, peanut butter, steak, cheesecake, and many non-healthy foods. Within just two weeks after my competition, I made sure I ate everything on that list. I didn't get sick, surprisingly, but I did put on weight—and fast. Within two weeks, I had gone from 10 percent body fat to 18 percent.

My first visit to my nutritionist post-competition was interesting. She suggested it was my hormones causing the weight gain, but I was honest and confessed to her everything I had eaten. She looked at me and said, "Feel better?" I didn't feel better. Although 18 percent body fat was perfectly healthy, I couldn't help but feel uncomfortable and chunky since I put the weight on in a matter of two weeks. I had enjoyed being really lean. However, I knew being *that* lean for long was not healthy or realistic.

Even though I only was able to maintain 10 percent body fat for a couple of weeks, I noticed that all of my clothes fit perfectly, and I felt lean and confident. At 10 percent body fat, I was able to fit into a size two pair of jeans. I didn't even wear a size two in high school, so you can imagine my excitement and confidence. I had the body I had always wanted! It was time for me to find my new balance. It took me about a month of hard work in the gym and clean eating to get back to a place where I felt comfortable.

I started doing my morning cardio again and kept all my meals squeaky clean. I took a mental note never to do that to myself again. I wanted to be a fitness model and knew I needed to find a lean, happy medium where I felt great every day. I also wanted to be dependable for future modeling jobs and keep my body toned and healthy.

I decided that 14 to 16 percent body fat was a healthy place for me to be. I could indulge in a cheat meal every couple of weeks yet still maintain a lean physique. I have discovered that when you set the goal to compete, it's not just important to focus on the big day of walking on stage, but also where you want to be afterwards. I have met many competitors who struggle to find their balance as well. After having several competitions under my belt, I honestly feel like I am in a good place with finding my own balance.

I allow myself a "fun meal" after a show, then I wake up and eat clean the next day. This is what works best for me and keeps me happy with my body and mind. There is nothing worse than eating junk for a week or two, knowing it will take you several weeks before you feel comfortable again.

Chapter 7

RELATIONSHIPS AND NEGATIVITY

During my twelve weeks of training, I prayed more consistently to God than I ever had before. Up until that point, I would pray before bed or meals or whenever it was convenient, I suppose. I believe that God has a plan for each of us to come closer to Him; we just have to be open to the opportunity. Once I started training for competition, I found myself praying for discipline, motivation, strength, wisdom, and even for relationships that were fading.

You see, when I became focused on eating clean foods, it became obvious which relationships were built around partying and eating as entertainment. I still attended social functions, yet I was questioned on how one drink would hurt and derail me from my goals. It is one thing for someone to ask but to be ridiculed or criticized is entirely different. Eventually, I stopped being invited to dinner parties when I started bringing healthy dishes that were not covered in cheese and had fatty ingredients.

Honestly, I was pretty exhausted with the idea of defending or explaining myself at yet another event. It was very obvious who supported me and who did not. I don't believe that those people quit liking me as a person, but I just believe our interests changed. It was hard to understand why a handful of friends stuck by my side, supported, and encouraged me, yet others wanted nothing to do with my new lifestyle and went as far as to say they did not "agree with it." Some of the people I thought of as "friends" just flat out didn't even acknowledge or show interest in my new lifestyle and goals.

After talking with other people who have made this same lifestyle change, I realize that most of them have also dealt with negativity and people who don't understand their goals. At the end of the day, we are all human beings, and everyone fights some sort of battle. Why not support each other? I've learned that just because someone doesn't choose my path and I don't choose theirs, that doesn't make either of us wrong. We have simply found our own ways to accomplish what we want in life.

Once I discovered new (sober) ways to have fun, I really started enjoying a better quality of life. Not only did I enjoy still being social but I could also eat clean all week long and enjoy the results it brought my body. My workouts had once been a dreaded activity that brought little change and much frustration. Once I started eating clean, non-processed meals, I realized I had the key to creating the physique I wanted. I had never felt so alive and happy with my mind and body. I found myself being so thankful for the handful of loved ones who supported my new goals. They loved me for me, not just because I fit into their lifestyles.

This realization made me hold these loved ones even closer and cherish them more than ever. Today, I'm still the same Kelsey, only with more confidence, new leadership skills, a positive attitude, and a FIT body! Finding your passion can clear your mind and help you trim off the excess negativity very quickly. I have found that some people are threatened or envious of passion—not because they share your same goals necessarily, but because they just haven't found their own passion. They might wonder, "Who are you to have THAT goal?" The answer that I've found is, "Who are you NOT to have THAT goal?"

Also, when you are practicing strict self-discipline, it can cause others to look at themselves and wonder why they cannot do the same. The comfort I find in this idea is that those who love you will support your goals. If you are leading by example then you will have a positive influence on those who want to make a change. Those who are unhappy with themselves will either let you be a positive influence and bright light in their lives, or they will reject what you are doing and exude negativity.

I believe that God doesn't plant a passion or dream inside of you that He doesn't want there. As long as that passion or dream is for His will, He opens doors that show you the way to get there. People will come into your life for a reason then leave. I believe that God takes the negative out to make room for the positive. That has certainly been the case in my life with a handful of relationships. I am very thankful for my close support group that loves me and supports my goals. In turn, I support those that I love, even if they do not share my hobbies and beliefs.

I encourage you to take a good look around you and ask yourself if you are surrounded with those who support your goals. If not, you might want to bow out gracefully and open your life up to positive energy. Change can be painful at first, but you will soon see the path that The Man Upstairs wants you to follow. Be strong. Stand for something and be confident in your beliefs.

Although I love modeling and always thought that would be my dream job, it becomes more apparent every day that I am truly fulfilled by serving others and helping someone else find his or her way in this world. There is no other feeling like that of helping someone achieve that seemingly unattainable goal and not expecting a thing in return. To do something for someone who can never repay you—that's the good stuff. That is where the passion and fulfillment comes in life: by helping others. It gives you a sense of purpose and creates a legacy you are proud to leave behind.

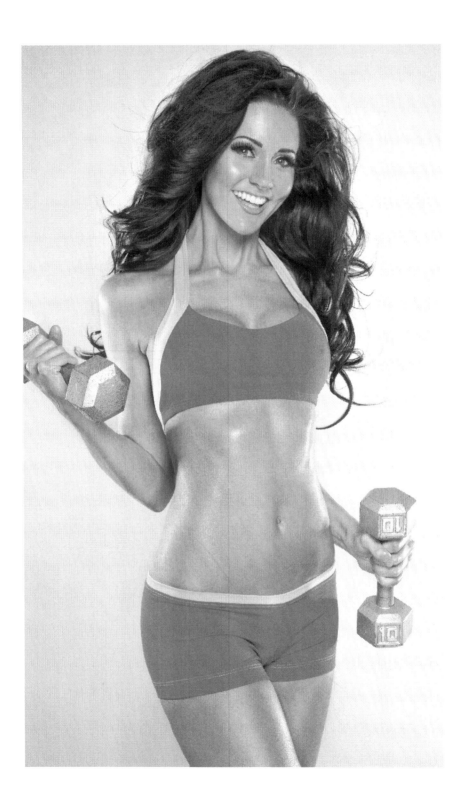

Chapter 8

FITNESS MODEL KELSEY

After my competition, my husband and I made the decision to let the year of 2011 be focused on developing my modeling portfolio. Once I was over the post-competition "pig out" phase, I focused on getting my body photo shoot ready again. I knew that 10 percent body fat was not a realistic goal, so I decided I felt healthiest at about 15 percent. This goal allowed me to stay lean and still enjoy an occasional cheat meal and more complex carbohydrates in my meal plan.

I had been following a certain photographer's work for three years at that point. I decided to save my money and book a shoot. This was another big step for me. I was still coming to grips with the fact that I had achieved my fitness goals for my body. I booked the shoot, which was out of state and completely outside of my comfort zone.

The shoot allowed me to gain experience in front of the camera and become more relaxed with posing. I believe you have to figure out which angles look best on-camera with your body. Practice makes perfect! That first photo shoot made me feel confident and beautiful. I was thrilled with the outcome of my photos. I decided I was interested in working with magazines to be published and have the opportunity to reach more people. I quickly scheduled a follow-up shoot with the photographer to expand my portfolio.

The second shoot was very successful. Out of those photos, I was soon published in nine magazines. I quickly figured out that in order to get published, it pays off to save your money and actually hire the photographers who work with the magazines. It doesn't guarantee that you will get published, but if the magazines like your look and you earn a good reputation in the industry, your chances of publication are very likely.

I also started to understand that fitness competitions and magazines are two completely different businesses. Of course, if you become a professional competitor, your chances of getting published in magazines are very likely. However, for the average bikini or figure competitor participating in local shows, you are not likely to get discovered by magazines. This was a reality check for me because when I took the stage for the first time, I was secretly hoping for exposure.

While competing did introduce me to a new form of discipline, it did not get me noticed by any magazines. It did, however, get me noticed by Labrada Nutrition and resulted in my becoming a sponsored athlete. If your goals are to compete, go pro, and get sponsored, I would recommend that you continue to work your hardest and compete. If your goals are to become a fitness model and get published, I would recommend focusing on your portfolio, working with the published photographers, and submitting your photos to magazines.

I also contacted a local modeling agency and sent in some snapshots my husband took with our camera. I signed a contract with the agency and started booking paid jobs for fitness advertisements. At one point, I felt like I was leading two separate lives. I would go to work full time, sitting behind a desk all day.

Then I would work part time as a model when I was booked for jobs. I started gearing more of my life toward fitness.

My outings with friends were planned around when I could get my workouts in. I wouldn't say I was obsessed; I just had new priorities. I decided I would need to stay in shape year round to be considered a dependable fitness model. This may sound silly but the first few months of actually referring to myself as a fitness model in conversations with others seemed strange. I finally decided it was an acceptable title once I started making money from my modeling jobs. I even started a public Facebook page and website to market myself as a fitness model and personality.

At first, I debated whether or not I should post my "chunky" photos from college. I was a bit humiliated that I ever let myself get that far off track. I took the page down several times and thought to myself that maybe that was too personal of a topic to put out there for the public to see. I also doubted that many people were interested in my posts and photos.

However, once I chickened out and took the page down, people started emailing me to ask about the page. Friends and family were passing the page on to motivate others trying to lose weight.

I started receiving emails from perfect strangers who told me that my photos had changed their lives. It was then that I knew I did the best thing by putting my embarrassing photos out there. Any bit of embarrassment I felt was far surpassed by the fulfillment of inspiring someone to make a positive lifestyle change. I decided then and there to be proud of where I'd been and what I had learned along the way. I haven't looked back since.

My public Facebook page grew surprisingly quickly. I posted motivational quotes and anything that inspired me. I also posted informational articles that I found on the topics of nutrition and working out. I wanted the page to be informative instead of all about me. I quickly discovered that my passion wasn't only modeling but helping others. I gained great fulfillment from answering emails from others just searching for a way to get healthy. I knew from experience how powerful and helpful one simple email could be.

Another turning point in my career as a fitness model was shooting with *Oxygen Magazine*. In January 2012, I made my goal to shoot with Oxygen, then I put my plan into action. My husband and I attended the Arnold Classic in Columbus, Ohio, in March 2012. Up to that point, I had followed the work of *Oxygen Magazine*'s photographer. I booked him for a photo shoot while we were in Columbus. I expressed my goals to him and explained that it was my career goal to shoot with him and *Oxygen Magazine*. I felt like the biggest nerd but at least I was honest.

Not only did we have a great shoot, he invited me to eat dinner that night with the entire *Oxygen Magazine* staff. I was in disbelief during dinner and knew that thousands of women would have loved to have been in my seat at that very moment. The *Oxygen Magazine* staff reviewed my photos and I was soon invited to travel to Canada to shoot for the magazine. Several months later, my ultimate dream came true.

Oxygen Magazine put me on their fall 2012 "Off the Couch" fat loss magazine cover! I was blown away. My cover came out just two years after I entered the fitness industry in my first bikini competition. Shooting with *Oxygen Magazine* was a career goal for me, as the publication was a big part of my motivation during my fat-loss journey. October 2012 was also a very important month because I launched my very first twelve-week challenge, sponsored by Lean Body for Her and Labrada Nutrition. I named it, appropriately, The Kelsey Byers Challenge.

I designed the challenge based on the foods I eat every week. I even provided a meal plan and workout plan for challengers. To my surprise, my challenge had over seven hundred participants. I was very pleased with the results and I am so proud of the ladies who put in the hard work to change their bodies and lifestyles.

So much of my life has become about motivating other people to make positive changes in their lives. I truly get my fulfillment from helping someone else who cannot possibly repay me. It is amazing what God will do in your life when you let Him take control. I used to stress so much about what my life should be. I wondered what my calling was.

Once I stepped back, eliminated negativity, and focused on me and my relationship with God, my mind became very clear. I made my health a priority and everything else fell into place. When you make your health your priority, everyone around you gets the best of you: your family, friends, work, school...the list goes on and on.

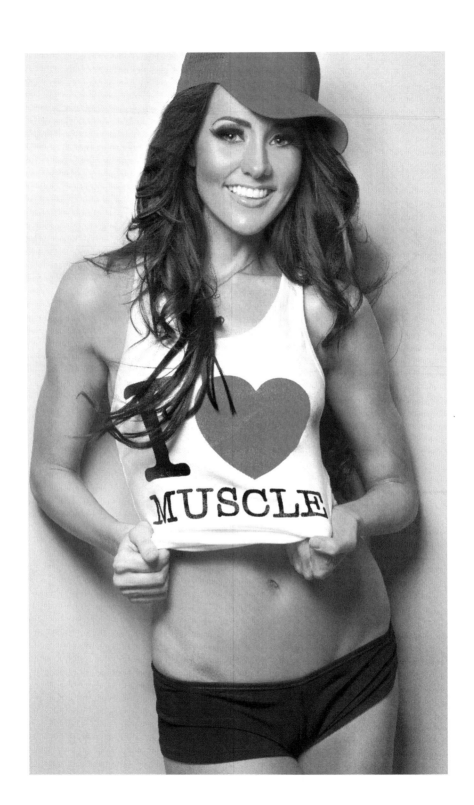

Chapter 9

THE NEXT STEP

Once I saw how I could achieve my goals by practicing self-discipline, I started focusing on other areas of my life. I started attending church regularly and taking on more projects at work. At the beginning of each year, I sit down and write out a list of goals I would like to accomplish, both short-term and long-term. It's surprising, but actually taking the time to write them out somehow makes them real.

I don't let myself get overwhelmed with long-term goals. I simply focus on the short-term ones a day at a time and make small steps toward accomplishing the long-term goals. I give myself a weekly "to-do" list, crossing out the tasks as I complete them. I plan out my workouts, meals, school assignments, modeling goals, and more.

If you have goals you want to achieve, I would recommend writing out weekly, monthly, and yearly plans. I find that it helps me stay focused. In today's world, it is really easy to get sucked into social media on a daily basis. In the past, I would sit down at the computer and, before I knew it, two hours had gone by.

I have found that if I force myself to accomplish certain tasks before sitting down at the computer for social networking, I am pleased with myself at the end of the day for having been productive. Don't forget: there is always someone getting a workout in while you are surfing the Internet. Set time aside for your personal goals and then use the time left to network, watch TV, or whatever you choose.

As you can see from my progress pictures, I am not an overnight success. It took me quite some time to make a habit of consistent clean eating and working out. Don't think you have to give up everything cold turkey. Ease into a healthy lifestyle. Make it enjoyable for you. Don't have the impression that it's ALL OR NOTHING. That's unrealistic.

Also, *decide* on your goals. Everyone's goals are their own and are different. My goals have changed over time. Nine years ago, I just wanted to avoid going out for fast food after going out with friends. Five years ago, I simply wanted to avoid drinking alcohol during the week and wanted to fit into size six pants. I did what I needed to do to achieve those goals, then I moved on to bigger ones. Now my goals mainly consist of being the healthiest I can be year round and reaching out to others to promote a healthy lifestyle. Therefore, everything I do is geared toward accomplishing this. That makes me the happiest Kelsey I can be!

This is YOUR life; live it at your own pace. Don't compare your progress to someone else's. Everyone's body is different and reacts differently to food and exercise. You see, from the outside, what looks like an "overnight success" is really a ton of small goals that led to one HUGE goal of earning and creating the body of my dreams, feeling healthy, and being HAPPY! It is actually what you do *when no one is looking* that counts the most. No one can stand over your shoulder and tell you, "Eat this, not that" or "You'd better go work out." YOU simply have to give yourself a million pep talks and remind yourself of your original goal and WHY you are doing this.

Chapter 10

MAINTENANCE AND CHEAT MEALS

In my journey, I have found that the "maintenance" of a fit body is fairly easy when I keep my meals clean. I find that it is realistic to stay lean year round by planning my meals and work-outs each week. My husband and I cook in bulk on Sunday and Wednesday. Occasionally, we will cook our meals for the week on Sunday and freeze some in Tupperware dishes. The preparation actually saves time over the course of a week because you aren't going to the grocery store and cooking. In turn, this gives you more time to work out, work on hobbies, and spend with your family.

The key is finding your healthy balance for your schedule. It's worth stepping outside your normal routine to try cooking in bulk. We thought it was different at first, but now it's just part of our normal routine as a family. We simply plan those nights for cooking our food and then we are free the rest of the week to accomplish what we want.

Another important factor when maintaining a healthy body and weight is your allowance of cheat meals. Like I said previously, I went on a "cheat meal" spree after my first competition, and I was not happy afterwards. As a result of my spree, I put weight on quickly and felt uncomfortable for about a month or two.

By making clean eating part of your lifestyle, you can look great all year and still enjoy a cheat meal here and there. For example, if I don't have a modeling job or an event coming up, I will allow myself a dinner or two out every couple of weeks. At dinner, I order whatever I want. Whether it is chips, salsa, guacamole, wine, or sushi, I eat the meal and don't feel guilty because, three hours later, I eat a clean meal.

My metabolism never slows down because I don't stop eating. I also only have one cheat meal. I don't have a cheat day. The worst thing you can do is indulge in a cheat meal and not eat anything the rest of the day. By not eating, you slow your metabolic rate, which causes you to gain weight over time. This hinders your progress, so I wouldn't advise it. By simply eating clean and enjoying an occasional cheat meal, I have not gained any of my college weight back. I have simply found a healthy balance for my life.

My definition of a cheat meal has certainly changed over the last few years. My husband and I used to have an entire cheat day. Whoa, it made us feel sick. Plus, we weren't getting the results we wanted, even though we worked out five to six days a week. Then we changed to a cheat meal every week and would go and get a burger with tater tots or go eat Mexican food. That would have been fine, only we weren't eating the right portions during the week, so we still didn't see the results we wanted.

Finally, we hired our nutritionist and cut our cheat meals back to once every two weeks. This saved us money from going out to eat and we quickly saw the results we wanted. These days, if I want something "cheat-like," it's frozen yogurt (fat-free with no sugar added) OR a couple of rice cakes with natural crunchy peanut butter OR sushi with brown rice. My version of a cheat meal didn't change overnight. By simply changing my habits, my cravings slowly changed.

When it comes down to it, when you can change the way you think about food, you CAN go without cheat meals. It's fuel, not entertainment or something to make you feel comforted when stressed. When I changed my view on food, my world completely changed. Your mind controls your body! At the end of the day, moderation is key. Find your balance so you don't feel restricted.

Chapter 11

CELLULITE

When I gained weight in college, my body stored a large amount of cellulite on my glutes and hamstrings. I never thought I would lose the cellulite and had lost all hope of having a beautiful backside and lean legs again. However, when I hired my nutritionist, she informed me that as my body fat decreased, my cellulite would, too. Hearing this little bit of information was the first hope I had found in years.

When training for my first bikini competition, I discovered that my cellulite disappears when I am just under 15 percent body fat. Any time I have had a few extra cheat meals and let my body fat rise over 15 percent, I develop this little dimple of cellulite on the back of my leg that I like to refer to as "Dimpsey."

Although Dimpsey alone isn't really enough cellulite to depress me, when he shows his ugly face, I know I need to quickly get refocused and clean up my meal plan. If you are facing problems with cellulite, just know that it is usually the last bit of fat to leave your body, so don't get discouraged. Consistent clean eating and exercising will reduce the amount of cellulite. Just be patient and put in the hard work. It is so worth it!

Chapter 12

ALCOHOL

I'm often asked the question, "Do you drink?" I drank when I was chunky. I was chunky when I drank. Both are true. Alcoholic beverages contain sugar alcohol. When I drink, it hinders muscle growth and I hold on to extra fat. It doesn't matter what kind of alcohol I drink: beer, vodka, wine, etc. None of it helps me accomplish my goals. So, when I decided to get healthy and drop the weight, alcohol was the first bad habit I kicked. Don't get me wrong: I have a past of ordering yummy margaritas at dinner, but I also was not proud of my body then. Drinking normally leads to snacking, which cancels out my hard work in the gym.

I do like to have a glass of wine occasionally, but when I do, I try to limit it to one glass. In the end, this is your life and you should enjoy yourself. Take everything in moderation. Quite honestly, I would rather have a good cup of coffee over wine these days. I got over the drinking kick once I discovered that alcohol leads to cellulite. I knew it had to go.

If you love to have your wine or refreshing adult beverage, I would advise limiting it to the weekend only while you are trying to lose weight. One of my first major changes in my body happened when I cut out drinking alcohol for one month during my college years. It was difficult being in social settings, but I pulled it off. I dropped at least five pounds that month just from avoiding alcohol. My clothes fit better and I felt great. For best results with fat loss, I would advise limiting your alcohol consumption. However, for tips on fitting your beverage of choice into your meal plan for moderation, I would advise hiring a nutritionist to help you out.

Chapter 13

SLEEP AND WATER

Two factors that affect your ability to lose weight are your water intake and the amount of sleep you get. Your muscles grow when you are resting, so plenty of sleep will aid in muscle repair and keep your energy levels high. I aim at getting seven to eight hours of sleep per night.

I have noticed that by keeping my body hydrated, I don't have any problems shedding weight. Drinking plenty of water also keeps me feeling full until my next meal. If you are concerned that you are not drinking enough water, you should consult with your doctor or nutritionist.

In the past, I have made the mistake of thinking I was hungry when really I was just dehydrated. Don't confuse the two. I have gotten my best results from eating a non-processed meal every three hours and drinking plenty of water throughout the day. As far as other liquids, I will have a cup of coffee in the morning with fat-free, sugar-free powdered creamer. I have a glass of green tea every other day. Green tea is loaded with antioxidants and it keeps my skin and hair looking healthy.

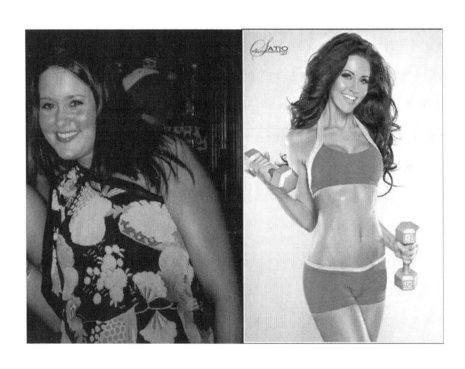

Chapter 14

WORKING OUT

When I first started lifting, I'm pretty sure I began with five-pound dumbbells. I quickly learned that I should be challenged by that last set, otherwise I was lifting too light, which means no change. My husband reassured me in the beginning that since I am a woman, I don't have the testosterone needed to build bulky muscle that most women are afraid of. Once I realized that I would not bulk up, I stopped being afraid of lifting heavy. It was then that I got my best results. My body started to transform its shape, creating a nice and fit package.

As a rule, I usually stick to completing three sets of eight to twelve on upper body and four sets of twelve to twenty for lower body. I choose three to four exercises per muscle group and work out each muscle group per week. If I choose to do an extra day, I work out my weakest area twice, waiting three days in between workouts. For example, I might choose to work out my glutes on Tuesday and then again on Friday.

One of the most common questions I get is, "How do I know when to increase my weight?" If I'm doing military press for my shoulders and lift twenty-pound dumbbells, I will do three sets of eight for this workout. That last set of eight should be tough.

The next week when I do shoulders again, I do three sets of ten. The next week, three sets of twelve. Then I'm at the point where I will increase my weight to twenty-five-pound dumbbells. I keep a notebook to track all of my weights. If I feel like I just can't increase anymore on a particular exercise, I pick a new exercise for that muscle group.

It's normal to feel your muscles burn during a workout and be sore the following day or two after lifting. If not, pick up some heavier weights to challenge yourself. The goal with lifting is to concentrate on slow, controlled movements. Unless you are over-eating, you will not put on fat by lifting weights. By hiring a nutritionist, you will find out that there are certain meal plans that are best for building muscle and others that are best for getting lean. They key is to find the perfect balance to meet your goals.

This is where eating clean becomes so important. You want to be sure you are fueling your muscles; otherwise, your body won't change. That was the point when my husband and I hired our nutritionist. We felt sluggish in the gym and wanted to fuel or bodies to finish our workouts strong. I usually lift weights for two muscle groups per workout. The following is my schedule for lifting weights and cardio:

I like to do cardio three to four mornings a week on an empty stomach. I prefer steady-state cardio, such as the elliptical, stairmill, or walking uphill on the treadmill. Every other day, I will incorporate some HIIT (high-intensity interval training) by adding a forty-second sprint (with no incline) every ten minutes of walking uphill on the treadmill. This keeps my heart rate up and has proven very effective when I'm trying to shed fat. I would recommend working out your most stubborn area twice in one week.

Weight Schedule:
Monday: Shoulders and abs
Tuesday: Legs and glutes
Wednesday: Rest

Thursday: Chest and triceps
Friday: Back and biceps
Saturday: Optional—legs and glutes, day two
Sunday: Rest

Chapter 15

BALANCING THE LIFESTYLE

I have met many people throughout my fitness journey. Many struggle with finding their perfect balance among fitness, life, fun, and fitting it all in. I believe it's important to realize that no one can be perfect 100 percent of the time. No one has the perfect schedule. Life happens. Your plans and schedule can get derailed.

There are family functions, weddings, parties, and plenty of other opportunities to miss a meal or eat something off of your clean meal plan. That's okay. To me, the idea is to have more "ON" days than "OFF" days. I try to eat as clean as I can during the week and on the weekends that my husband and I don't travel. That way, I can save my "cheat meal" for a special occasion.

This balance is a key factor to my success as a fitness model and feeling great in my own skin year round. The summer is usually the easiest season for me to stick to my clean meals 99.9 percent of the time. There are plenty of opportunities to be in a swimsuit, and I always want to feel my best. However, once the holidays roll around, I find myself a little more laidback with my meal plan when it comes to social gatherings with family and friends. You have to enjoy life, right?

I have been known to sneak a clean meal into a Thanksgiving or Christmas dinner, though. I believe it's important to have healthy options around, even if I want to sample other dishes as well. During the holidays, I make sure I don't miss my workouts since I know I'm more likely to have a few more cheat meals than the norm. I try to limit myself to one cheat meal per week during the holidays.

You don't want to end up regretting your decisions when January comes around. I like to make my New Year's resolutions about goals other than losing weight, so I keep my meals as clean as possible during the holidays.

Chapter 16

FINDING YOUR MOTIVATION

When looking for motivation, keep in mind that the beginning of your weight loss journey is the hardest. It is easy to get frustrated because you may be working really hard in the gym and you may be eating super clean, but, in reality, the results are not instant. I remember that it took my body a good two to three months of clean eating to show big results. You have got to trust the process and fuel your body with the proper food to support an active lifestyle.

Throughout my journey and especially in the beginning, I relied on my favorite fitness magazines and photos of my favorite athletes for motivation. I made a "focus" bulletin board with photos of bikini competitors and motivating quotes to keep myself on track. I put the board in a location that I saw every day, like my home office. I even started a folder on my computer of photos of fit women who inspired me.

The motivation ideas worked because I eventually saw my own awesome results. You have to find what makes YOU tick!

Don't let photos of athletes depress you; let them drive you. If they can do it, so can you! Trust me, if you stick to a consistent plan of eating clean and working out, your own results will start motivating you. There is nothing like waking up in the morning to new progress. There is no other satisfaction like knowing you gave the day everything you had and took more steps toward your goals.

If you are comparing your body to someone else's, make sure you have similar body types. There are plenty of athletes I admire, but I don't beat myself up over not having a body like someone who is five-three. I am tall and it is hard for my body to hold muscle. Therefore, if I choose to benchmark my progress based on someone else's physique, I make sure we have similar body types before comparing. Keep in mind, no one is made exactly how you are. Given the proper nutrition and training, your results could eventually be even better than the person you are admiring.

I encourage you to look at my progress photos and understand that my results did not come overnight. My weight loss was a gradual process because I did not understand what a significant impact nutrition would have on my outcome. If I had realized it sooner, my weight loss would have happened in a matter of months versus years. Still, I am thankful for my entire journey and the lessons I've learned along the way.

No matter where you are in your own fitness journey, appreciate every step and document the process. Take progress pictures and measurements every two to four weeks. If not for photos, I would not know today how far I've really come. People look at me now and never know that I was in a size fourteen just a few short years ago. If not for photos, there would be no way to inspire others in the same situation. There would be no proof that anyone can change their thoughts about food and alcohol and make a life change.

Chapter 17

EATING CLEAN

Here's the good part! My definition of eating clean is: eating a non-processed meal every three hours. Here is a list of foods I eat every week. This will help you get started eating clean. I hired my nutritionist to help me determine proper portions to meet my goals. The portions change when my goal changes—for example, my meal plan varies depending on whether I am training for a competition or just maintaining a healthy weight. Eating measured portions has helped me achieve the body of my dreams. I also like the thought of knowing I can eat everything on my plate without over- or under-eating. If you are ready to take your body to the next level, it may be worth hiring a nutritionist to help you. I understand that it is not in everyone's budget to hire a nutritionist right away, but I suggest saving and investing in your body, at least until you know how to do it yourself.

I eat every three hours, five to seven meals per day. This keeps my metabolism high and allows me to burn fat efficiently. Once I realized this and started practicing clean eating, I started seeing REAL results. As a rule, I choose a lean protein, complex carbohydrate, and veggie at each meal. These are "safe," generic portions to use in order to practice portion control and avoid overeating:

PROTEIN = Handful size
COMPLEX CARB = Fist size
VEGGIE = Two handfuls
FATS = Small, cupped palm size

*Note: These are foods I eat on a weekly basis. This can serve as a guideline for you. If you have food allergies or certain preferences, you may want to consult with a doctor or nutritionist.

PROTEIN:
Extra-lean ground turkey or tenderloin
Chicken breast or tenders
Fish (tilapia, shrimp, or Mahi)
Egg whites
Extra-lean beef
Fat-free cottage cheese
Tofu
Greek yogurt

COMPLEX CARBS:
Oatmeal
Grits
Brown rice
Whole-wheat bread or Ezekiel bread
Beans
Corn or wheat tortillas
Edamame
Low-sodium rice cakes
Yams
Potatoes
Fruit

VEGGIES:
Fresh or frozen vegetables are acceptable.
Asparagus
Green beans
Squash
Zucchini
Salad—with fat-free dressing
Spinach
Cucumbers

*Note: There are many more vegetables you can eat, so just check out your produce section at your local store.

HEALTHY FATS:
For healthy fats, I usually have one or two a day, eating them later in the day when my carbohydrates are lower in portion size. Again, this is where a nutritionist's customized plan for your body will come in handy. It is very important that you don't overeat so you don't store the extra as fat.

Examples of healthy fats include:
Avocado
Olive oil
Almonds, cashews, or walnuts
Natural peanut butter

FRUIT:
Treat fruit as a carbohydrate. It would be a great meal if you pair it with Greek yogurt or other lean protein source. I usually limit fruit to one meal a day to avoid extra sugar.

STAPLES:
I love to season my food with Mrs. Dash's salt-free seasoning, salsa, spicy mustard, low-sugar marinades, etc. You really just

have to get creative with it! My husband and I cook with fat-free cooking spray, but we use it sparingly.

SUGAR:

I avoid alcohol since it hinders my progress. I drink water or green tea.

As far as your sugar intake, I would recommend keeping it around or under about thirty to thirty-five grams per day, not counting sugar found naturally in fruits or vegetables. Sugar can add up fast and eating or drinking too much of it may be keeping you from meeting your goals.

Chapter 18

GETTING STARTED

The first step to getting started is to identify your goals. That's easy, right? I believe there are many people out there who say they have goals yet don't have a daily action plan to complete them. I would recommend making a five-year plan. What would you like to accomplish in five years? That may seem like a good distance in the future, but it will be here before you know it. Your plan can be for any type of goals for health, fitness, relationships, faith, school, career, you name it. Start here:

MY FIVE-YEAR PLAN IS:

_____

_____

_____

_____

_____

_____

_____

_____

_____

_____

_____

Next, write out a yearly plan. Specify steps you will take each month or each quarter to move toward those goals.

Years ago, my mom and I decided to write our New Year's resolutions on note cards. We each kept our note cards on our bedside tables to look at each night before bed, then we would review them again each morning. This concept keeps your goals on your mind and keeps you focused. I still do that to this day. I constantly surround myself with notes and reminders that keep my "eyes on the prize," whatever that may be. Writing out a yearly plan gives you twelve months to plot out your steps, moving closer and closer to that five-year goal. It is important to put your written goals in a place where you will see them each day. I recommend making a focus board/bulletin board, or keeping a notebook or journal.

MY ONE-YEAR PLAN IS:

_____

_____

_____

_____

_____

_____

_____

_____

The next step is to write out a monthly and weekly plan. For example, if you know you want to lose ten pounds in two months, plan out your meals and workouts for a few weeks at a time. Identify which days you plan to go grocery shopping and cook in bulk for the week. Plan your workouts as well. Sure, schedules can change, but having a plan in place is better than not having one at all.

I find that when I put my meal planning and workouts first after family priorities, my tasks always get done. When I put them off and take care of everything else in the world first, they don't get my full attention and I don't set myself up for success. That can result in missing meals and workouts.

MY MONTHLY PLAN IS:

_____

_____

_____

_____

_____

_____

_____

_____

_____

_____

_____

MY WEEKLY PLAN IS:

_____

_____

_____

_____

_____

_____

_____

_____

_____

_____

It would be beneficial to buy a planner to schedule your workouts and meals. Some people choose to use their smart phones to track their schedules. There are many apps today that will track your meals and workouts. Personally, I still get excited once a year to go to an office supply store and buy my yearly planner. There is something about having my plans in writing that makes it "real" or "official." Plus, I don't have to worry about the battery dying. I always have access to my planner, no matter what.

Chapter 19

QUICK TIPS FOR BEGINNERS

- Eat a small meal, consisting of a lean protein and complex carbohydrate, every three hours, five to seven meals a day.

- Drink plenty of water.

- Get plenty of rest; seven to eight hours of sleep per night.

- Start lifting weights; engage in cardiovascular activity (three to five days a week).

- Avoid fast food and fried food, and limit alcoholic beverages.

- Track your workouts in a journal.

- Write out your goals.

- Make a "focus" bulletin board to keep in a place where you'll see it daily; attach positive quotes, pictures and goals.

- Try new activities each week so you don't get bored. For example, try an actual workout class to keep you moving.

- Workout with a partner to hold yourself accountable.

- Surround yourself with positive people.

- Keep a planner to journal your daily meals.

- Believe in yourself! If you can convince your mind, you can do anything.

CLOSING

Thank you for taking an interest in my fitness journey and healthy lifestyle tips. I am happy to write this book because I know it would have helped change my life just a few years ago. It's amazing how you can change your path when you light that fire of determination. You have to *decide* you are ready. There is no person who can do it for you. I challenge you to give your body just two to three months of clean eating. What have you got to lose? Just remember, the "fun foods" will always be there later.

Don't feel like you have to quit your old habits cold turkey; just ease into the new lifestyle. I would start by eating a small meal every three hours. I did not become a fitness model, sponsored athlete, and motivated individual overnight. It took me a few years to ease into what I now consider "normal."

I invite you to continue following my journey through my website, blog and social networking. I love responding to your questions, so please contact me with any successes, struggles, questions, or thoughts that you may have.

How long should you eat clean? Well, it all depends on how long you want to look and feel great! It's not about a diet—it's a LIFESTYLE change. Just remember: eat clean and follow your dreams!

.

INSPIRATIONAL MESSAGES

During my fitness journey, I have received so many inspirational emails. I keep a folder of those that really make a difference in my day. If I think I'm having a rough time or things just don't seem to be going right, I read my emails. It completely turns my mood around and brings a big smile to my face! Thank YOU to everyone who has taken time out of their day to brighten mine with a message. You really don't know how much of a difference you are making!

"Thank you so much for all of the encouragement and tips on how to proceed in this new venture. Your advice is irreplaceable and I couldn't ask for a better person to have as a mentor! Thank you again for all of your help and motivation through all of this. Your advice and encouragement mean the world to me!"—Tiffani

"I feel the need to thank you, times a million. I truly can't tell you how thankful I am to have you as my inspiration. I have currently lost seventeen pounds and 5 percent body fat, all thanks to you. In three months' time, I have lost the weight and body fat by clean eating, lifting weights, and cardio. You have changed my life forever, and I know a lot of other people have been touched by you as well. You will continue to be my inspiration and motivation. Thank you so much!"—Andrea

"Kelsey, I just want you to know how much you inspire me and say a big thank you! I was introduced to you through the *Oxygen Magazine* article and soon after found your fan page. I appreciate and admire your honesty and sincerity; it's nice to see that someone with so much success is still 'normal.' Your progress pictures floored me and it hit me: 'I can do this!' You have had a huge impact on my daily workout and diet, so much so that I have sent your pictures to my trainer and nutritionist as the goal look. Best of luck and thank you!"—Virginia

"You're officially INTERNATIONAL! Congrats, Kelsey, this is awesome! Two years ago you were just Kelsey Byers from a little Texas town and now you are in a European magazine! I can't wait to see what will happen in five years! This is a dream come true for you and I'm so happy for what you have been blessed with. You made this happen! Your persistence and drive made your dreams come true and you have inspired so many women to pursue their dreams. It is one thing accomplishing a dream, but to inspire others is the greatest reward! Congrats!"—Roxanna

"Hey, Kelsey! Just wanted to tell you that a couple of my students stopped by my office and noticed your before/after pictures and quote that I have on my desk. They couldn't believe you were once that girl. One of them said, and I quote, 'If SHE can do it, anyone can!!' The quote I have posted is: 'The thing is, if you tell yourself you will NEVER have a fit and healthy body, then you won't. If you DECIDE to make a positive change and have that determination and discipline, you WILL make the change you desire!' Just call me the next Kelsey Byers. :) That's MY goal. Thank you for being such an inspiration!! I look forward to your daily tips and posts."—Jennifer

"Thank you for being so honest and genuinely interested in teaching/helping others. You have truly changed my life. God bless you and I wish you all the success in the world."—Kim

"I just wanted to say THANK YOU for putting up your BodySpace and transformation. YOU ARE MY INSPIRATION to be a better person. You kept your diet and workout simple and I appreciate that. A lot of them are very confusing. YOU have a great body and congrats on succeeding with your dream. I hope you continue to inspire people and keep your dreams a reality. People like you make it possible for others! Thank you, Kelsey, from the bottom of my heart. Keep rockin' it, girl."—Karolina

"I have to admit there were times that your posts on Facebook annoyed me. Don't worry: it was only because I was mad at myself! I was jealous! Finally, your posts got to my head. I am only happy now when I work out and eat clean! How crazy! I hated it—now I love it. I check your Facebook page, when in doubt, to motivate myself. Now, thanks to you, it is time to get rid of unwanted fat and make myself strong! I will definitely wear your wristband all of the time! No excuses! Thank you so much for: your Facebook page, positivity, posting pictures of you (it helps to visualize my goal!). You look so strong! I love it! And, finally, thank you for being an amazing and motivating role model."—Olivia

"Hi, Kelsey. I had emailed you around a month ago about contact information on Kim Porterfield. You were so kind and replied, and I made a phone appointment with her. I finally had my appointment with her this past Wednesday and I am just so excited! I just had to share this with you... One of the initial questions she asked me was, 'What is your goal?' My response: **'Well, my inspiration is your client Kelsey Byers.'** Kim's response was, 'I couldn't be happier that Kelsey is your inspiration because she is the sweetest, most caring girl that I have ever come across.' I write this with nothing but appreciation for sharing part of your life with so many others, including myself. I have been an avid exerciser for years now but I would keep sabotaging myself with moments of binging on unhealthy food choices and probably lack of carbs, among not eating every three hours. Therefore, I'm not getting the results with all the hard work I put in at the gym. Regardless, there are not many people like you who share what you do in hopes of motivating and inspiring others. Again, thank you for wanting others to be successful in their fitness journeys!"—Lisa

"I have to thank you for, first, the motivational wristband and, more importantly, for sharing your entire story with the world. Thank you for proving that it **CAN** be done. You keep me motivated even when it feels hopeless and inspire me not to settle. Best to you!"—Emily

"Thank you for being the body transformation model for Bodybuilding.com. My fifteen-year-old daughter and I have been struggling to find a way to help her get her fitness under control for the past year. Reading your story made it seem so much more feasible. She felt so encouraged this morning that we are trying to 'restart' her program. What an inspiration you are!"—Debbie

THE END

24796706R00054

Made in the USA
Lexington, KY
01 August 2013